This Book Belongs To

Name: ....

Address: ....

....

....

....

Tel: ....

Email: ....

Notes: ....

....

....

....

....

....

....

....

Pet Type:

Breed:

Date of Birth:

Gender:

Weight:

Date	Age	Vaccine	Yet

Notes:

_____

_____

_____

_____

_____

Pet Type:

Breed:	Date of Birth:

Gender:	Weight:

Date	Age	Vaccine	Yet

Notes:

_____

_____

_____

_____

_____

Pet Type:

Breed:

Date of Birth:

Gender:

Weight:

Date	Age	Vaccine	Yet

Notes:

_____

_____

_____

_____

_____

Pet Type:

Breed:

Date of Birth:

Gender:

Weight:

Date	Age	Vaccine	Yet

Notes:

Pet Type:

Breed:

Date of Birth:

Gender:

Weight:

Date	Age	Vaccine	Yet

Notes:

_____

_____

_____

_____

_____

Pet Type:

Breed:

Date of Birth:

Gender:

Weight:

Date	Age	Vaccine	Yet

Notes:

Pet Type:

Breed:

Date of Birth:

Gender:

Weight:

Date	Age	Vaccine	Yet

Notes:

_____

_____

_____

_____

_____

Pet Type:

Breed:	Date of Birth:

Gender:	Weight:

Date	Age	Vaccine	Yet

Notes:

_____

_____

_____

_____

_____

Pet Type:

Breed:

Date of Birth:

Gender:

Weight:

Date	Age	Vaccine	Yet

Notes:

_____

_____

_____

_____

_____

Pet Type:			

Breed:	Date of Birth:

Gender:	Weight:

Date	Age	Vaccine	Yet

Notes:

_____

_____

_____

_____

_____

Pet Type:

Breed:

Date of Birth:

Gender:

Weight:

Date	Age	Vaccine	Yet

Notes:

_____

_____

_____

_____

_____

Pet Type:

Breed:

Date of Birth:

Gender:

Weight:

Date	Age	Vaccine	Yet

Notes:

_____

_____

_____

_____

_____

Pet Type:

Breed:

Date of Birth:

Gender:

Weight:

Date	Age	Vaccine	Yet

Notes:

_____

_____

_____

_____

_____

Pet Type:			

Breed:		Date of Birth:	

Gender:		Weight:	

Date	Age	Vaccine	Yet

Notes:

_____

_____

_____

_____

_____

Pet Type:

Breed: **Date of Birth:**

Gender: **Weight:**

Date	Age	Vaccine	Yet

Notes:

_____

_____

_____

_____

_____

Pet Type:

Breed: | **Date of Birth:**

Gender: | **Weight:**

Date	Age	Vaccine	Yet

Notes:

Pet Type:

Breed:

Date of Birth:

Gender:

Weight:

Date	Age	Vaccine	Yet

Notes:

_____

_____

_____

_____

_____

Pet Type:

Breed:

Date of Birth:

Gender:

Weight:

Date	Age	Vaccine	Yet

Notes:

Pet Type:

Breed: **Date of Birth:**

Gender: **Weight:**

Date	Age	Vaccine	Yet

Notes:

_____

_____

_____

_____

_____

Pet Type:

Breed:

Date of Birth:

Gender:

Weight:

Date	Age	Vaccine	Yet

Notes:

_____

_____

_____

_____

_____

Pet Type:

Breed: **Date of Birth:**

Gender: **Weight:**

Date	Age	Vaccine	Yet

Notes:

_____

_____

_____

_____

_____

Pet Type:

Breed:

Date of Birth:

Gender:

Weight:

Date	Age	Vaccine	Yet

Notes:

_____

_____

_____

_____

_____

Pet Type:

Breed:

Date of Birth:

Gender:

Weight:

Date	Age	Vaccine	Yet

Notes:

_____

_____

_____

_____

_____

Pet Type:

Breed:

Date of Birth:

Gender:

Weight:

Date	Age	Vaccine	Yet

Notes:

Pet Type:

Breed:

Date of Birth:

Gender:

Weight:

Date	Age	Vaccine	Yet

Notes:

Pet Type:

Breed:

Date of Birth:

Gender:

Weight:

Date	Age	Vaccine	Yet

Notes:

_____

_____

_____

_____

_____

Pet Type:

Breed:

Date of Birth:

Gender:

Weight:

Date	Age	Vaccine	Yet

Notes:

Pet Type:			

Breed:		Date of Birth:

Gender:		Weight:

Date	Age	Vaccine	Yet

Notes:

_____

_____

_____

_____

_____

Pet Type:

Breed:	Date of Birth:

Gender:	Weight:

Date	Age	Vaccine	Yet

Notes:

_____

_____

_____

_____

_____

Pet Type:

Breed: **Date of Birth:**

Gender: **Weight:**

Date	Age	Vaccine	Yet

Notes:

_____

_____

_____

_____

_____

Pet Type:

Breed:

Date of Birth:

Gender:

Weight:

Date	Age	Vaccine	Yet

Notes:

Pet Type:

Breed:

Date of Birth:

Gender:

Weight:

Date	Age	Vaccine	Yet

Notes:

_____

_____

_____

_____

_____

Pet Type:

Breed: **Date of Birth:**

Gender: **Weight:**

Date	Age	Vaccine	Yet

Notes:

_____

_____

_____

_____

_____

Pet Type:

Breed:

Date of Birth:

Gender:

Weight:

Date	Age	Vaccine	Yet

Notes:

_____

_____

_____

_____

_____

Pet Type:

Breed:

Date of Birth:

Gender:

Weight:

Date	Age	Vaccine	Yet

Notes:

_____

_____

_____

_____

_____

Pet Type:			

Breed:		Date of Birth:

Gender:		Weight:

Date	Age	Vaccine	Yet

Notes:

_____

_____

_____

_____

_____

Pet Type:

Breed:

Date of Birth:

Gender:

Weight:

Date	Age	Vaccine	Yet

Notes:

Pet Type:			

Breed:		Date of Birth:	

Gender:		Weight:	

Date	Age	Vaccine	Yet

Notes:

_____

_____

_____

_____

_____

Pet Type:

Breed:

Date of Birth:

Gender:

Weight:

Date	Age	Vaccine	Yet

Notes:

_____

_____

_____

_____

_____

Pet Type:

Breed:

Date of Birth:

Gender:

Weight:

Date	Age	Vaccine	Yet

Notes:

_____

_____

_____

_____

_____

Pet Type:

Breed:

Date of Birth:

Gender:

Weight:

Date	Age	Vaccine	Yet

Notes:

Pet Type:

Breed:

Date of Birth:

Gender:

Weight:

Date	Age	Vaccine	Yet

Notes:

Pet Type:

Breed:

Date of Birth:

Gender:

Weight:

Date	Age	Vaccine	Yet

Notes:

_____

_____

_____

_____

_____

Pet Type:

Breed:

Date of Birth:

Gender:

Weight:

Date	Age	Vaccine	Yet

Notes:

Pet Type:

Breed:

Date of Birth:

Gender:

Weight:

Date	Age	Vaccine	Yet

Notes:

_____

_____

_____

_____

_____

Pet Type:			

Breed:		Date of Birth:	

Gender:		Weight:	

Date	Age	Vaccine	Yet

Notes:

_____

_____

_____

_____

_____

Pet Type:

Breed:

Date of Birth:

Gender:

Weight:

Date	Age	Vaccine	Yet

Notes:

Pet Type:

Breed:

Date of Birth:

Gender:

Weight:

Date	Age	Vaccine	Yet

Notes:

_____

_____

_____

_____

_____

Pet Type:

Breed:	Date of Birth:

Gender:	Weight:

Date	Age	Vaccine	Yet

Notes:

Pet Type:

Breed:

Date of Birth:

Gender:

Weight:

Date	Age	Vaccine	Yet

Notes:

_____

_____

_____

_____

_____

Pet Type:

Breed:	Date of Birth:

Gender:	Weight:

Date	Age	Vaccine	Yet

Notes:

_____

_____

_____

_____

_____

Pet Type:

Breed:	Date of Birth:

Gender:	Weight:

Date	Age	Vaccine	Yet

Notes:

_____

_____

_____

_____

_____

Pet Type:

Breed:	Date of Birth:

Gender:	Weight:

Date	Age	Vaccine	Yet

Notes:

_____

_____

_____

_____

_____

Pet Type:

Breed:

Date of Birth:

Gender:

Weight:

Date	Age	Vaccine	Yet

Notes:

Pet Type:

Breed:

Date of Birth:

Gender:

Weight:

Date	Age	Vaccine	Yet

Notes:

_____

_____

_____

_____

_____

Pet Type:

Breed:

Date of Birth:

Gender:

Weight:

Date	Age	Vaccine	Yet

Notes:

_____

_____

_____

_____

_____

Pet Type:

Breed:

Date of Birth:

Gender:

Weight:

Date	Age	Vaccine	Yet

Notes:

_____

_____

_____

_____

_____

Pet Type:

Breed: | **Date of Birth:**

Gender: | **Weight:**

Date	Age	Vaccine	Yet

Notes:

Pet Type:

Breed:

Date of Birth:

Gender:

Weight:

Date	Age	Vaccine	Yet

Notes:

Pet Type:

Breed:

Date of Birth:

Gender:

Weight:

Date	Age	Vaccine	Yet

Notes:

_____

_____

_____

_____

_____

Pet Type:

Breed:

Date of Birth:

Gender:

Weight:

Date	Age	Vaccine	Yet

Notes:

_____

_____

_____

_____

Pet Type:

Breed:

Date of Birth:

Gender:

Weight:

Date	Age	Vaccine	Yet

Notes:

Pet Type:

Breed:

Date of Birth:

Gender:

Weight:

Date	Age	Vaccine	Yet

Notes:

Pet Type:			

Breed: | **Date of Birth:**

Gender: | **Weight:**

Date	Age	Vaccine	Yet

Notes:

_____

_____

_____

_____

_____

Pet Type:			

Breed:		Date of Birth:

Gender:		Weight:

Date	Age	Vaccine	Yet

Notes:

_____

_____

_____

_____

_____

Pet Type:

Breed:

Date of Birth:

Gender:

Weight:

Date	Age	Vaccine	Yet

Notes:

_____

_____

_____

_____

_____

Pet Type:

Breed:

Date of Birth:

Gender:

Weight:

Date	Age	Vaccine	Yet

Notes:

_____

_____

_____

_____

_____

Pet Type:

Breed:

Date of Birth:

Gender:

Weight:

Date	Age	Vaccine	Yet

Notes:

_____

_____

_____

_____

_____

Pet Type:

Breed:

Date of Birth:

Gender:

Weight:

Date	Age	Vaccine	Yet

Notes:

Pet Type:

Breed:

Date of Birth:

Gender:

Weight:

Date	Age	Vaccine	Yet

Notes:

Pet Type:

Breed:	Date of Birth:

Gender:	Weight:

Date	Age	Vaccine	Yet

Notes:

_____

_____

_____

_____

_____

Pet Type:			

Breed:	Date of Birth:

Gender:	Weight:

Date	Age	Vaccine	Yet

Notes:

_____

_____

_____

_____

_____

Pet Type:			

Breed:	Date of Birth:

Gender:	Weight:

Date	Age	Vaccine	Yet

Notes:

Pet Type:

Breed:	Date of Birth:

Gender:	Weight:

Date	Age	Vaccine	Yet

Notes:

_____

_____

_____

_____

_____

Pet Type:

Breed:	Date of Birth:

Gender:	Weight:

Date	Age	Vaccine	Yet

Notes:

Pet Type:

Breed:

Date of Birth:

Gender:

Weight:

Date	Age	Vaccine	Yet

Notes:

Pet Type:

Breed:	Date of Birth:

Gender:	Weight:

Date	Age	Vaccine	Yet

Notes:

Pet Type:

Breed:

Date of Birth:

Gender:

Weight:

Date	Age	Vaccine	Yet

Notes:

_____

_____

_____

_____

_____

Pet Type:

Breed:	Date of Birth:

Gender:	Weight:

Date	Age	Vaccine	Yet

Notes:

Pet Type:			

Breed:		Date of Birth:

Gender:		Weight:

Date	Age	Vaccine	Yet

Notes:
_____
_____
_____
_____
_____

Pet Type:			

Breed:		Date of Birth:	

Gender:		Weight:	

Date	Age	Vaccine	Yet

Notes:

Pet Type:			

Breed:	Date of Birth:

Gender:	Weight:

Date	Age	Vaccine	Yet

Notes:

_____

_____

_____

_____

_____

Pet Type:

Breed:	Date of Birth:

Gender:	Weight:

Date	Age	Vaccine	Yet

Notes:

_____

_____

_____

_____

_____

Pet Type:			

Breed:		Date of Birth:	

Gender:		Weight:	

Date	Age	Vaccine	Yet

Notes:

_____

_____

_____

_____

_____

Pet Type:

Breed: **Date of Birth:**

Gender: **Weight:**

Date	Age	Vaccine	Yet

Notes:

_____

_____

_____

_____

_____

Pet Type:

Breed:

Date of Birth:

Gender:

Weight:

Date	Age	Vaccine	Yet

Notes:

Pet Type:

Breed:	Date of Birth:

Gender:	Weight:

Date	Age	Vaccine	Yet

Notes:

Pet Type:

Breed:

Date of Birth:

Gender:

Weight:

Date	Age	Vaccine	Yet

Notes:

Pet Type:

Breed: **Date of Birth:**

Gender: **Weight:**

Date	Age	Vaccine	Yet

Notes:

Pet Type:

Breed:

Date of Birth:

Gender:

Weight:

Date	Age	Vaccine	Yet

Notes:

_____

_____

_____

_____

_____

Pet Type:

Breed: **Date of Birth:**

Gender: **Weight:**

Date	Age	Vaccine	Yet

Notes:

_____

_____

_____

_____

Pet Type:

Breed:

Date of Birth:

Gender:

Weight:

Date	Age	Vaccine	Yet

Notes:

_____

_____

_____

_____

_____

Pet Type:

Breed:	Date of Birth:

Gender:	Weight:

Date	Age	Vaccine	Yet

Notes:

Pet Type:			

Breed:	Date of Birth:

Gender:	Weight:

Date	Age	Vaccine	Yet

Notes:

_____

_____

_____

_____

_____

Pet Type:

Breed:	Date of Birth:

Gender:	Weight:

Date	Age	Vaccine	Yet

Notes:

_____

_____

_____

_____

_____

Pet Type:

Breed:

Date of Birth:

Gender:

Weight:

Date	Age	Vaccine	Yet

Notes:

Pet Type:

Breed:	Date of Birth:

Gender:	Weight:

Date	Age	Vaccine	Yet

Notes:

Pet Type:			

Breed:		Date of Birth:	

Gender:		Weight:	

Date	Age	Vaccine	Yet

Notes:

_____

_____

_____

_____

_____

Pet Type:

Breed:

Date of Birth:

Gender:

Weight:

Date	Age	Vaccine	Yet

Notes:

Pet Type:			

Breed:		Date of Birth:	

Gender:		Weight:	

Date	Age	Vaccine	Yet

Notes:

_____

_____

_____

_____

_____

Pet Type:

Breed:	Date of Birth:

Gender:	Weight:

Date	Age	Vaccine	Yet

Notes:

_____

_____

_____

_____

_____

Pet Type:			

Breed:	Date of Birth:

Gender:	Weight:

Date	Age	Vaccine	Yet

Notes:

_____

_____

_____

_____

_____

Pet Type:

Breed:

Date of Birth:

Gender:

Weight:

Date	Age	Vaccine	Yet

Notes:

Pet Type:

Breed:	Date of Birth:

Gender:	Weight:

Date	Age	Vaccine	Yet

Notes:

_____

_____

_____

_____

_____

Pet Type:

Breed:	Date of Birth:

Gender:	Weight:

Date	Age	Vaccine	Yet

Notes:

_____

_____

_____

_____

_____

Pet Type:

Breed:	Date of Birth:

Gender:	Weight:

Date	Age	Vaccine	Yet

Notes:

_____

_____

_____

_____

_____

Pet Type:

Breed:	Date of Birth:

Gender:	Weight:

Date	Age	Vaccine	Yet

Notes:

Pet Type:			

Breed: **Date of Birth:**

Gender: **Weight:**

Date	Age	Vaccine	Yet

Notes:

_____

_____

_____

_____

_____

Pet Type:

Breed:

Date of Birth:

Gender:

Weight:

Date	Age	Vaccine	Yet

Notes:

Pet Type:

Breed:	Date of Birth:

Gender:	Weight:

Date	Age	Vaccine	Yet

Notes:

_____

_____

_____

_____

_____

Pet Type:

Breed:

Date of Birth:

Gender:

Weight:

Date	Age	Vaccine	Yet

Notes:

Pet Type:

Breed:

Date of Birth:

Gender:

Weight:

Date	Age	Vaccine	Yet

Notes:

Pet Type:

Breed:	Date of Birth:

Gender:	Weight:

Date	Age	Vaccine	Yet

Notes:

Pet Type:

Breed:

Date of Birth:

Gender:

Weight:

Date	Age	Vaccine	Yet

Notes:

_____

_____

_____

_____

_____

Pet Type:

Breed:

Date of Birth:

Gender:

Weight:

Date	Age	Vaccine	Yet

Notes:

_____

_____

_____

_____

_____

Pet Type:

Breed: **Date of Birth:**

Gender: **Weight:**

Date	Age	Vaccine	Yet

Notes:

Pet Type:

Breed:	Date of Birth:

Gender:	Weight:

Date	Age	Vaccine	Yet

Notes:

Pet Type:

Breed:

Date of Birth:

Gender:

Weight:

Date	Age	Vaccine	Yet

Notes:

_____

_____

_____

_____

_____

Pet Type:

Breed: | **Date of Birth:**

Gender: | **Weight:**

Date	Age	Vaccine	Yet

Notes:

Pet Type:			

Breed:		Date of Birth:	

Gender:		Weight:	

Date	Age	Vaccine	Yet

Notes:

_____

_____

_____

_____

_____